SLEEVER
XL to XS

A. Kavanagh

Copyright © 2019 Strategic Fund Ltd

All rights reserved.

ISBN:

DEDICATION

To Mum and Dad, your love and support has and always will be cherished everyday.

CONTENTS

	Acknowledgments	i
1	Had Enough	1
2	Undercover	Pg 11
3	Preparing	Pg 21
4	Touch Down	Pg 33
5	Surgery	Pg 43
6	Post	Pg 50
7	New Regime	Pg 59
8	Coping	Pg 72
9	New Life	Pg 88
10	Domino	Pg 92

ACKNOWLEDGMENTS

To all the Surgeons, Medical Staff and Hospitals, we thank you for this amazing life-saving surgery that changes the lives of those that would otherwise be rendered lost in a world of helpless struggle.

1 HAD ENOUGH

If you've started reading this book you are more than likely at your wits end with the scales. Perhaps you're strangely curious to find out what the real life journey of a middle aged bariatric sleever looks like. Whatever your motivation this book has captured an in depth real life perspective that's uniquely different. The journey along with all its pitfalls, triumphs and epic transformations make for essential reading for those seeking to embark on this type of surgery. Alternatively it can help you if you're fresh out of the operating theatre, with real examples of what worked and what to avoid. We hope by reading this sleever's journey you will learn from my personal mistakes and be inspired to achieve your dream dress size and move towards your own ideal weight, whatever you choose it to be. Believe it or not I'm pretty good at losing weight, I have done it more times than I choose to remember, yet somehow I would predictably end up gaining any weight I had lost and then some every single time. Who knows I'm probably much like you, I've been on every weight loss plan known to man, had the hypnoses, read the books, bought the treadmills, subscribed to the wonder pills and basically joined in on all the latest fads that've kicked around over the last 30 years. My problem was quite simple, every time I lost the weight my head told me I was finally at the pinnacle. I now felt what skinny felt like and boy was it good. At this point my brain told me I didn't need to watch what I ate any longer. (big mistake) I thought I was now cured. Truth is that I would never be cured without changing something bigger. This was a lifelong battle that required me to never release or relax and discard the healthy lifestyle. It always felt the same, almost like I had achieved a miracle, fought a hard battle and won. Yet every time I lost the weight I quickly put it straight back on again. I knew I needed a more permanent solution. When I occasionally achieved my happy place my unfunny husband would often joke with me thinking he was commending me on reaching my newest milestone and finally grasping that elusive goal weight. He would often chuckle... "So you've lost the weight eh, do you think you will be able to find it again?" he would then go into an uncontrollable laugh at his own misguided humour and disappear off before it got really ugly for him. Luckily for him, as he was about to choke if he hung around too much longer. Unfortunately there was always a way that I did manage to find it again, find it and some became the way things usually went. Over time I realised the voice inside my head was somehow working against me, I lacked the tenacity to persevere after the massive struggle to lose the weight. I would reach a point on the scales and feel pretty comfortable and somewhat content, this would in turn flood me with enough emotion to let go a little and relax the reins on my tightly regimented eating program. Just for a wee moment I would take the time to reflect on my new found awesomeness. This was enough to let bad habits get another foothold and left me open for another battle. And then in a few weeks I would wake up in what seems like a little more than an overnight slip up and I would be back to my now largest weight ever. Once again I'd be fighting desperately to stop gaining, before long I would be looking for a new eating regime whilst blaming the last one for its epic short comings. Weight gain and loss to me was a form of torture and somewhat like a rare disease, something that you had to learn to live with, sort of like an impairment only this one was unfortunately somewhat self-imposed. Yes it appeared that I could change to get a better life, yet I couldn't really cure myself completely. It just kept coming back to haunt me time and time again, to beat me to the ground and remind me that I was never going to be in control. I thought a lot about finding another way, and if there was one what could I do to end the unending madness? Was I different from the rest of society? probably not, as it seems everyone's fighting the same battle in some form or another. Yet this girl wasn't getting any wins. At times I totally wanted to give it up and live my final days as an overweight stay indoors middle aged wife. Hopefully that would help me have everlasting happiness. But deep down behind the coca cola and mud cake I didn't want to be a loser. It seemed counterfeit to give up without a decent fight, but could I fight any harder? Could I actually win this battle? To make things worse it was obvious to me that if I didn't tackle this it could seep into other areas of my busy life, like a persistent problem it would eventually negatively impact on my career, social engagements and even our family leisure activities. I couldn't give up and settle, it just wasn't right. My husband tried to convince me from time to time in his normal salesy way that he wanted a different life for me, I guess he could also see that the door was closing on things that we could both enjoy, like hiking, biking or just spending time together outside of the four walls of home. He feared in the long run that he would probably be doing these things alone, and that scared him. Especially if I couldn't win the food war. He got desperate and even rejigged the Def Leopard song "Poison" cheekily singing it when I poured another Coca Cola, it was his way of reminding me of the effect the sugar was having on my well rounded body, well as you can guess that didn't work much either, so I did what anyone would do when their husband doesn't agree with their choices, I doubled down. I figured that I needed a solution that would end my wasted life battle once and for all. So I toyed with the idea of having some form of weight loss surgery. There was so much to consider though, quality of life post op, would I enjoy food anymore, and what about the inflated medical costs. Then there were other questions like where would I have the surgery and would it actually be effective on me. In my mind the time to do something about it was most definitely now. I felt that any longer and I'd be too old, too fat or too deep in my ways to change. Let's start with a little background about me and our life, Two years ago I was in my late forties part Maori, part European. married and reasonably active and let's face it, large. As a married couple we had recently become empty nesters with our son completing his hard earned Law degree, we were on the other side of things, at a brand new crossroad in our lives. So we mused for hours about what the future would actually look like now that there was just the two of us alone at home. I was still a Mum that's for sure but the dependent dynamics of our sons relationship had just changed, and this self-confessed "smother" had to step away somewhat quietly. Hubby sensing a vacuum and the flood of emotions that would follow started talking about what our awesome child-independent future might look like, emphasising that it probably included some sort of exotic travel which by the way would require me to squeeze into one of those ridiculously tiny plane seats. He even kidded that we would be laying around on those busy tourist beaches with a bathing suit on or if he was choosing a bikini. You think it might've dawned on him that my body didn't belong on any beach and that this was one of my biggest fears, nope not a chance not him. I mean I love that he accepts me unconditionally whatever my shape is that week, but hubby is an ocean loving, occasional surfer that needs to be outdoors to enjoy the elements. He got so excited with the possibilities of this new found life that he even suggested relocating to the beautiful beaches of sunny Gold Coast where its bloody warmer for a lot longer than the average NZ summer, and by at least three months! Panic flooded my mind and my head played that classic horror music before someone is about to die. What was this slightly obese wife and mother of one going to do? I was desperately trying to figure out how to derail the dreams of my mate of 34 years and let him down gently and simply because I'd let things go without getting a handle on my weight, wow I let that sink in. Reality was making me uncomfortable and I slowly began to realise that there was no way I could possibly enjoy a future journey with the man I love just because I couldn't accept my overly critical self image. Yes I was large and some people would tell me to get over it, there are lots of people that are large and still manage to live life to the full. It seems that some girls have no problem whatever their size, unfortunately I'm not one of them. However I processed it I felt deeply aware that this newly found freedom would ultimately come adrift. I was sadly at a point where I had become aware of just how much damage I'd done. I really did not recognise who I saw in the mirror and sadly in my head I was still that 16 year old on my first date. It's at this stage that you ask yourself those tough questions, like how in God's name did I get here? One minute I'm admired, next minute I'm invisible. Sure we should age gracefully and some admittedly do a better job of it than others. Me well I'd broken the golden rule in ageing gracefully I'd clearly not looked after myself and had fast approached the point of no return. Believe me that is a really tough lesson, to think that you can't reboot your life and come back from it can look a little dire indeed. The pain that I was feeling at this time most people would call reality, its a place that I found was much easier to ignore than to receive feedback from. I stopped weighing or measuring myself for this very reason and found shops with large fitting small sizes to further confuse my reality. It was sometimes just too much for me to cope with, it felt like there was no way of stopping and that the walls were closing in on me. So I decided that change needed to happen. Having tried and failed this doom loop so often, it appeared that the only way to control a food demon was a full on exorcism by a catholic priest or a visit from Jesus himself. Luckily there was light at the end of this dark night, a new day could come my way by removing most of my ever demanding stomach. It seemed like a pretty drastic measure that's true but I had literally reached the end of a very wide road. I guess I'd finally "had enough" either surrender and cauterise the problem or die unchanged and feeling I never reached my potential. This war needed to be stopped before I stopped caring. I knew there was a better life void of uncontrollable cravings and it was waiting for me on the other side of a surgery door somewhere out there, I just knew it.....

2 UNDERCOVER

So I did what every well adjusted girl with a plan would do, I went full bore into a self-imposed and seriously covert research program. Partly because I cared what people would think about my medical assistance being a cop out and partly because I wanted to be fully armed with the most accurate information available. Eventually I would need to present a succinct argument on why this path was the best option for us and would hopefully be negotiating with my hubby on how to fund the surgery. Look let's be realistic I was totally confident I could persuade him, hell, he never said no to me about anything. But there were some tiny cracks in my reasoning that really needed addressing, these cracks could potentially affect our relationship. For instance, he will be uneasy and concerned that there's the possibility of death from complications on the operating table. Its thoughts like this that I needed to be armed with to combat his interrogation. So anecdotal information that would reassure him that I was signing us up for a robust and safe procedure would be critical. Then there's those hefty medical costs to consider, choosing one of the many available options could prove to be quite expensive. Let's face it this was both of our hard earned cash, many years of working, making a few mistakes, clocking up a few wins and owning a few things. Yet here I was selfishly wanting to spend a chunk of capital on fixing myself, and that seemed inherently wrong. I had obviously neglected myself for a long time and that was my fault, now it was going to cost both of us to fix it. Fortunately we would agree it needed to be done. The first operation on my radar was the gastric band it was the cheapest option by far and could be reversed if necessary. Which made it appear like a no brainer, affordable, reversible and effective. Yet unbelievably in the back of my mind that little voice was starting to harass me into thinking I could actually lose the weight have the band removed and voila I would be cured of obesity. Seriously looking back on this procedure now it was plainly unrealistic. I needed a more permanent solution anything less would prove to be a waste of time and money. To make matters worse I had discovered a family member who'd already had this procedure undertaken and admitted there was little success. As it turns out there is a small maintenance port placed on your skin to routinely tighten the band around the stomach which must be performed by a doctor. That alone seems wrong but in her case the band wasn't maintained and had little to no effect, so probably not the best example for me to base a decision on but it also was not a good option if we were to travel. I soon decided this procedure was not a contender for me. So I moved my search onto a Gastric Bypass, from one end of the spectrum to the other I guess. A small band to total removal of a functioning stomach, that'll do it I thought. You have more than likely experienced yourself that there is way too much information out there on these subjects. There were those that were pro bypass surgery singing their unique tunes and then the nay sayer's trying to sway you away. Some appear to be authorities having never had the surgery others are just not helpful enduring long rants about nothing. So sifting through the endless information had ultimately rendered me paralysed. I wasted far too much time listening to every side, eventually I gave it away and was more confused than a modern day voter trying to decide on a political spectrum. Fortunately ten years prior to my writing this book my mother successfully undertook Gastric Bypass surgery. These days the procedure is quite different to the original operation, as mentioned I had to do my own research to see if it was applicable. At the time the family forced an intervention as we all felt her health was slipping away. We decided the best way to help her at that time was a stomach bypass, if she would agree that is. Had we not put that plan together to help her there's a good chance that she wouldn't be with us today. In our minds it just had to be an option to consider. Mum thankfully agreed and in a short time after her surgery she went from a size 28 to a size 12 and at her smallest she reached a size 8! I was lucky enough to observe my mother's transformational journey and totally believed my future would probably mirror hers with the same drastic measure to curb my food cravings. She is such a strong woman, she never once let on that the first few years were so difficult, adjusting to her new stomach was tougher than I could ever imagine, every time we visited her we couldn't believe just how much weight had literally melted away from her, she looked amazing and interestingly her personality changed along with her shape. She was clearly far happier, wanted to socialise more and had become a clothes shopaholic. For the first time in her life she was proud of her new image. After she had lost a significant amount of weight she spoke about the way people had treated her when she was a larger woman and how things had changed now that she was smaller. It was apparent that years of weight directed sneers had obviously affected her pretty deeply, so much so that she eventually became a little negative and mostly defensive about everything. That thankfully all changed after the surgery and now she lives a great life and as Dad says they live in a "small drinking village with a fishing problem". Behind the scenes though, she could not tolerate a lot of foods, for instance any form of meat, bread or vegetables, her portion sizes were and still are teeny tiny, a couple of bites and she's done! Dumping [food does not agree with you and you immediately need to vomit] is horrendous for her which would occur after most meals she would instantly feel nauseated and have to run off to the bathroom to be sick. It would take so much out of her that most of the time you would not see her until the next day, as she would need that much sleep to recover. A word of warning... The food addiction that we have can sometimes shift effortlessly across to other addictions such as alcohol, gambling and shopping especially it seems with such drastic change. This became an actual thing, she had replaced eating food with shopping for all manner of clothes, more than likely because she felt great and at the time of writing her wardrobe is literally over flowing! I knew I also needed help with portion control but let's be realistic I still wanted to be able to taste the food and enjoy what little precious bites I could have. So I guess in a way my mum showed me through her own tough experience that this was definitely not the procedure for me, I would need to find an alternative if I was ever going to lose weight and remain sane. Luckily for me in that time a new weight loss procedure was developed, which lead me to accidentally coming across a gastric sleeve operation one night in one of my many online search marathons. And as it was fairly new to the market, it seemed that the techniques were still being perfected which in turn made me a little nervous. Interestingly this procedure quickly became the number one weight loss choice within a few short years. Basically the operation consists of some form of reduction as the surgeon removes 75-80% of the stomach through a few very small incisions in the abdominal wall, (in my case three) he then stitches the stomach closed and sends you onto recovery and then later to heal in a general ward for five days, starting back with a soup diet. You essentially receive the stomach you had as small child, which leaves you nervous about the lack of sustenance and a fear that you could burst the stitches if you over ate, vomited or even drunk coca cola ever again. This knowledge alone will turn your appetite off severely. I remember at this point getting pretty excited and must've binge watched every You tube video ever made about the subject, from gastric sleever's, doctors and clinics. Some were upbeat and informative others not so much, each one though had me hooked a little more. I remember coming across one awesome lady that cemented me in. She was close in age to me and had video'd herself the day before her procedure, then again the day after and then every month after that for the next 8 months. She was nothing short of inspiring she shared her struggles her win's and her immense progress. Of course every time I logged in her lovely face popped up and there she was shrinking before my very eyes.

I was sold. I wasn't afraid of the procedure anymore and just wanted it done as soon as possible. Once again my inner voice reminded me of my worst fear, what if I lost the weight was it possible I could find it again (thanks for that hubby, what a winner). From what I had researched there were a few that had actually regained their weight. I mean my head was now spinning how is that even possible? Some more research produced the answers and I found that apparently you could stretch your stomach all over again if you made bad food choices - that is fizzy drinks, sugar, or even excess carbohydrates. It dawned on me that this may not be the magic fix I thought it was. It now required that I needed to make good food decisions. Something I clearly was not accomplished at. I mean now I was really struggling, was this for me or not? I soon realised that this surgery gave you the tools to help with portion control not a guarantee for evermore, in a way it would reset my life to an earlier time and train me to eat like I should've up until now. Oh boy the dread set in, would I actually fail at this too? Either way win or lose, I felt I had no other real options, so I decided to go for it regardless of the outcome. Who knows I thought I could probably learn how to eat better even if it was for a short time. Little did I know at the time that this was not going to be a problem for me at all. This was definitely a tough point though, one that I was never going to tell the hubby about in my elevator sales pitch. For this operation to happen it required a water tight case, one that didn't involve regaining weight. Too bad though a few months later the Surgeon met with me us the night before the surgery and explained in minute detail that this operation could be undone by a complete lack of self-control and some easily made poor diet choices. The colour drained from my husband's poor face, he looked horrified and made the Doctor repeat the dialogue while he listened intently and later admitted at that point he wanted to up sticks, open the door and head for the hills!

3 PREPARING

I have always claimed that I would never make it in a sales career. It appears that I'm probably wrong on that assumption. I found it really can be boiled down to one key ingredient which is best described as "desperation" and now I was about to present my toughest pitch ever. This was the pitch that could change everything and I so badly needed to enjoy a healthier future for the many years to come. I set the scene by adding on a few more pounds, one of my easier implemented gifts in this life. Hubby and I sat down together at the dinner table to go over the plea for becoming thinner. I began by mentioning my lack of self-control and reminding him of my previous failings.

That once again I was out of doable options all the while gently coaxing him towards my latest idea. "I have found a way to live with lasting weight change and a way of protecting our sanity, how good is that?" I said in a reassuring tone. Marching on I pulled out all the stops, I made a promise that once I lost the weight I would have no trouble going to the beach and swimming with him. They say you need a winning close to seal the deal, so I reminded hubby of our families history of obesity, heart failure, diabetes and high blood pressure. On and on I ploughed forth with irrefutable arguments to justify the surgical risks that would finally remedy my potential ailments once and for all, at that point I knew he was onboard. As I mentioned earlier I was well aware that I would have hubby's support but it still felt right to make this decision together. After all there where risks and I knew I would absolutely need his emotional and physical support on the other side of the operating doors. Having hubby by my side through the recovery process and on to the complete retraining of my eating habits, was much easier. I strongly believe I couldn't have done anywhere near as well without his support. We agreed to proceed to the next level, my immediate task at this point was to report back on the costs and timing. It looked like this dream was starting to become a reality. The very next morning I picked up the phone and called a local Gastric sleeve surgeon for pricing, I must admit I was beyond excited, if they could wheel me in to surgery that afternoon I would've packed a bag and booked an Uber! Unfortunately my happy bubble would soon burst as the receptionist informed me that these operations would cost in the vicinity of $28K NZD and in addition would require a one night's stay in the hospital. I was also informed I would have to go on a liquid diet (sadly not wine) which consists of a meal replacement drink three times a day for three weeks prior to surgery to help shrink the liver. I desperately called two other clinics to compare prices and yep they were exactly the same. I banged away at my computer searching for cheaper options pouring over gastric sleeve sites until finally what should pop up on my search? A beacon of hope by way of advertisement for gastric sleeve surgery in Thailand. It was almost a third of the price, "yes we have a winner" I thought. I know what you're thinking, are they really even Doctors? What's the hygiene standard of those Thai hospitals like anyway? After all it is a third world country right? And like the rumours will I be missing certain body parts if I indeed even woke up from the surgery? My imagination ran wild. To be honest I was so ready to have this procedure the nagging doubts soon disappeared from my mind and over the horizon for me at least was that the reward outweighed the risk by a country mile. It didn't faze me one little bit, however I knew this would be a problem for hubby. Then there was my immediate family to consider, those who I would be confiding in. They would all probably try and stop me anyway. So once again I knew I would have to research everything thoroughly, regarding doctor, hospital and after care so at least I could make an attempt to combat the serious objections that were coming my way. There were a few companies organising medical tourism to Thailand throughout New

Zealand and Australia. Fortunately I was able to watch plenty of testimonies from happy Gastric Sleevers complete with before and after pictures. You could even privately message former patients and ask all sorts of weird questions which was amazing. I made contact with a lovely lady that lived 15mins from me that had been through the whole process, she was nothing short of inspirational, sharing with me her food battles what was working for her, what to avoid and she even went into great depth about how well she was looked after in Thailand. Thankfully she was a nurse in New Zealand and contrasted the two countries in detail for me... In New Zealand it would be a one night stay, Thailand was five nights in a hospital room that was more like a hotel suite. The Doctors and nurses were professional and always attentive in Thailand. She could not fault the pre op or the post op after care at all and that's from a medical professional. So once again I was sold, now to sell it to my hubby and family, that was definitely not going to be so easy. The correspondence immediately commenced between myself and a Thailand representative, it became clear pretty quickly that another major hurdle was coming my way. I was informed that I would need a medical check list signed off by my G.P. in New Zealand. Basically they were checking for sleep apnea, blood pressure and pre-existing conditions before they could consider me for the operation. Dread now filled me, this was a substantial hurdle for me overcome. You see my Doctor was an amazing man who by the way I had been going to see for more than 30 years, who knew my most intimate things, whom I trusted with my life and who had never let me down and was a straight up no nonsense sort of guy. In my mind there was no way this was going to fly he was not going to approve of me running off to Thailand for this operation and would want me to have it done right here in New Zealand. This was starting to get very real, I had made up my mind to go to Thailand no matter what anyone said. So I bit the bullet and started telling my loved ones of my plans, as expected hubby was not impressed with Thailand and our son was also not having a bar of it, he thought I had gone mad. "What is wrong with you Mum, have you lost your mind?" he exclaimed "You don't even need an operation, you're not that big!" Really are you serious son?" is all I could say to him along with "I don't need your permission, I was just letting you know out of courtesy!" I told hubby and disapproving son that there was one small hurdle to overcome and that was the final sign off from our Doctor. A wide smile formed across our sons face, his expression said it all. There was no way our Doctor would sign off, and he knew it, so he wanted front row seats to watch me be told a definitive no. "Mum I'm coming with you to see the Doc, I want to make sure you don't leave any details out when you're speaking to him." Wow how supportive my baby boy was being. I know the attitude came from a place of love but I felt like no one was in my Thailand corner, my Mum and Dad were all for the operation but definitely not in Thailand. They were encouraging me to have it done locally, and my baby sister got angry at me and said I didn't even need an operation, I wasn't that big, and did I realise I would probably die on the operating table or wake up missing body parts. She can be a little direct at times, don't get me wrong we are as close as two sisters can be. We adore each other, but she was rightly concerned and persuading me to rethink. My Brother surprised me though, he said "Good on you Sis, I know you've struggled with this for years so go for it!" I tell you that was heartwarming in a sea of negativity. I made my Doctors appointment for the very next day, and was anticipating his resistance which made me extremely nervous. That night I worried myself to sleep as I didn't want this journey over before it even began. True to my sons word he accompanied me the next day, joyful he was not. With all the emotion swirling around in the car on the trip out to the doctors I finally stepped up and said in my motherly authoritative voice, "If the Doctor gives me his blessing, you must back off and be supportive son, you got it!" he just cracked a smile and said "Sure Mum there's no way our Doc is signing you off, ever." The moment of truth finally arrived, here I was sat with my son beside me in front of my Doctor, "How can I help?" he asked a little curious as to why I had a young family member that by the way he had helped bring into this world, accompanying me. With a lot of apprehension the words came out of my mouth like a child in front of the headmaster, "I am thinking of going to get a... (nervous pause) Gastric Sleeve in Thailand and need your sign off to be able to proceed." I couldn't make eye contact with him at all and if I were standing I would've probably been shuffling uncontrollably. Time seemed to grind to a halt and stand still, the anticipation was by now really building. Strangely he asked me "What hospital are you looking at?" and "Who is the surgeon?". I remember thinking, now that's bloody weird why is he asking that? Well someone was watching over me, particularly on this decision because as it turns out my Doctor is on the board for a medical insurance company that arranges top end overseas care to reduce their claim expenses. They were doing the same as me I guess, trying to save a few bucks. He manages multiple procedures and Thailand was one of the countries he was directly involved in. So he said he would use his vast contacts to check out both the hospital and surgeon and then get back to me with his recommendations. He also reiterated that Thailand had some of the world's best surgeons and that the hospitals and equipment used is often superior to ours. As long as it was one of his known choices he would have no problem with me electing to have the procedure done overseas, and was also excited for me knowing my struggles with weight throughout my lifetime. Wow, just wow! To say I was happy was an understatement, relieved, ecstatic, euphoric would better describe my mood. I was considered defeated but not now, the discovery that my very own Doctor could research something this important for my family was nothing short of miraculous. Needless to say my son wasn't smiling anymore as we headed back home. The very next day my email dinged and there it was my Doctor confirming both the hospital and the surgeon were world class in gastric sleeve surgery. He had absolutely no hesitation in recommending them and wished me the best of luck! With signed off paperwork for Thailand, it was now game on! This little bit of information seemed to put my hubby and parents at ease. Now for the formalities, we just needed to decide when, how to pay for it and what to do while I recuperated. It wasn't as easy as picking a date at this point as hubby and I had made other life changing decisions too, we were selling the house and everything in it, The plan was to change everything and relocate to Queensland, Australia. If I was going to change I thought we might as well make it a big deal. We had no contacts or family there and we would be leaving our son in an apartment back in New Zealand, which broke our hearts into a million pieces. As you can guess I could write a book on how that was for me, I really had no clue when I painstakingly gave birth to him just how difficult enduring the day your child leaves the nest would be. Fortunately there is some joy being a Mum as you admire how they too learn to make massive decisions in their own life and head along the path to fulfilling their very own dreams. We decided that as soon as the house was sold we would book for Thailand and then on completing the recommended three week post op care we would fly straight into Queensland to begin our new adventure. Searching for a home and finding jobs would be top of our list. It would be such an upheaval, new city new stomach new jobs and new eating habits, epic changes that's for sure, and we were up for the challenge....

4 TOUCH DOWN

Things somehow went to plan, we had by now sold the house and decided to spend the last days with my parents prior to embarking on the "new me" journey. We moved our remaining possessions into one of their wardrobes and kicked around the drinking village for a while. By this stage we had secured a surgery date, paid the deposit and booked our flights. I was fully anticipating the end of my food woes, which sort of felt like a load had been lifted from my shoulders, with the added calmness of knowing things were about to change for the better. It was the pace of change to come that was far beyond anyone's expectation. We packed pretty lightly for the trip and I'd figured out that the clothes that I owned would be (if all went well) rendered useless within a few short months. I was pleasantly proven right on that hunch, but that said I still needed to pack in my trusted GHD hair straightener, rather large hairdryer and face care ensemble. So my bag was pretty light for a girl but nothing like hubby's who thinks it's a competition. He aims to board the plane with his number ones on and a throw bag with his number twos stuffed inside just in case something unusual should arise. The day finally arrived, so our parents thankfully drove us up the three hours to the airport, after we said our emotional goodbyes we set off to change me forever. Once we were onboard I started to ponder deeply as I weaved my way through those endless plane movies. I thought about what it would be like to never obsess about food again, or whether I could actually follow the dietary rules to ensure I wouldn't damage my new and improved stomach - Me version 2.0. Apparently as I've been told on many occasions I can be a bit of a broken arrow when it comes to both dietary rules and healthy food choices, but this was going to be mandatory portion control at the least. We'd taken an overnight flight thinking it was the easier way to sleep through the cramped seating arrangements and ultimately arrive refreshed. Unfortunately for me there was far too much on my mind and sleep wasn't one of them. By the time we landed in Bangkok I'd been awake for 22 odd hours, with a bit more to come as I would soon discover. We disembarked and made it to the customs line fairly quickly having only packed carry on luggage, unfortunately when we got there we couldn't make out the other end of the line as it snaked for what looked like a kilometre. About half an hour in some poor Asian lady pulled out a phone to take a photo and was pounced upon by a 5ft uniformed guard yelling "No photo!" and proceeded to threaten her with the back of the line. Good grief some people with power, who can figure that one out it's an enigma to me. After standing in line for over an hour and the usual processing we were exhaustedly out the other side. We had been given explicitly detailed instructions on pickup in an email, so we headed to find our collection point and clearly not too alert from all the sleep deprivation. Unfortunately we walked straight on past our names and off into the abyss. After much searching we realised we had no clue of what to do and succumbed to calling the representative who we had of course woken from a deep sleep. We were informed that the driver had left already thinking we didn't actually make it to the plane. He kindly turned around and headed back to collect us along with the other passengers that were waiting for us to find the pick up point (sorry Sonny). The driver finally got us to the hotel thirty mins later. We settled in and had the best sleep ever. From this experience we vowed that we would never again take a night flight if we could at all help it. The morning broke and we opened our sleep deprived eyes and those sound proof curtains on the awesome busyness that is Bangkok. It felt good to finally be here. Yet there was a nagging thought constantly jabbing me in the back of my mind. I was being reminded of what was about to descend on me, sort of like the beeping of a forklift in reverse before finally running you over. We headed down to the buffet to get in amongst it, which by all accounts was substantial. After breakfast and gratefully satisfied we decided to relax for the rest of the day to get a handle on our jet lag. Hopefully I would be rendered as fresh as possible for the appointment the following day. By the afternoon we had recovered sufficiently enough to go exploring and totally keen to hit the malls of this amazing city. Hubby had been here before for work so he was a bit like a tour guide with the added bonus of being able to speak really clear english. He got us on the back of two scooters as pillion passengers and headed us into MBK for a waffle washed down with a fresh mango smoothie. A note to self; don't let life pass you by without experiencing a scooter in Bangkok traffic, it was seriously scary yet strangely addictive. I'm sure I left my nails in some poor drivers bicep! As it was my first time here I was awe struck by the endless concrete structures and occasional vibrant greenery scattered randomly throughout, then there were the neon lights and the familiar smells of charcoal fired cooking. It also occurred to me that there was a massive financial divide between street vendors and their entrepreneurship selling all sorts of wares from food to trinkets and then the upper end hotels that cater for swathes of tourists from across the globe. Bangkok was truly an eye opener, my only hope was that the hospital was more like the hotels than the street vendors, if it was the other way around I would more than likely be heading back home in a few days. We made it back after dinner and set in for the night anticipating the next day's events. I was scheduled to meet the Surgeon for the first time face to face. As planned we were picked up from the hotel and taken to the hospital which geographically was not that far maybe six kilometres or thereabouts, but once you factor in the traffic thirty five mins later we arrived. We were immediately ushered through to a private reception area for sleevers and the likes. This is where the agency leased an area inside the hospital that housed the support nurses and customer service staff who worked busily on the countries biggest earner known fondly as

"Medical Tourism". There were a contingent of nurses that tended to us in small rooms checking our weight, blood pressure and the likes, one nurse in particular was absolutely stunning inside and out, she explained in great detail how renowned my surgeon was and how he had performed thousands of these procedures with nothing short of stellar results. Basically I was in the best hands available. The nurse also made a bold prediction she said "When you come back here, the day before you leave for your final examination you will be down at least 10 kg's!" No way I thought as great as that sounded my mind could not comprehend it, I just smiled. It was quite a sight to observe all the goings on, the pick ups and drop offs, the patients shuffling in at various stages of repair or for the hastier walkers more than likely being admitted. The largest groups were from New Zealand and Australia. At that time most of us were there for Sleeve surgery and the rest were there for a variety of cosmetic surgeries most popular being face lifts and mummy makeovers after sleeving. The next book goes into detail covering my experience with skin removal along with all the learnings and procedures. But here we sat comparing our food battles and stories all the while recommending to each other where to go for the best shopping, nicest food and how not to get ripped as a fresh tourist. There was undoubtedly a great camaraderie between us all, a place where lasting friendships would be born and journeys shared over the years to come. Before too long my beautiful representative appeared before me and informed me that my surgeon had just arrived. She ushered me on towards the examination room where I would meet him for the first time. My mind was swirling with questions. Who was this man, what was he like and could he be the one that changed me forever. I entered the consultation room and there he was my modern day saviour, he was a handsome man, gracefully kind, smiley and super friendly, typical of a lot of the Thai people we met on this trip. I remember him instantly putting me at ease, he firmly shook my hand and invited me to take a seat. I realised fairly quickly that he had a pretty decent sense of humour, as he cheekily said

"So you've had enough now?" I didn't quite understand maybe it was the broken english or I was so nervous that my brain had vacated the room for a moment. I looked at him confused by his question, so he tried a different one "You want to now live a longer better life?" "Yes, yes I do!" I stammered finally comprehending his questions. "Yes Doctor, I have had enough!" I replied "Very good, now you have to work hard, I will shrink your stomach but you must change your food and drink habits," he looked to gain my commitment saying "Do you think you can do this?" My head was pretty much saying probably not, but my mouth confirmed the words he wanted to hear so I blurted out "Yes I can!" He explained that I would lose approximately 60% of my excess weight. For me that would calculate out to about 60% of my 40kgs excess, equating to about 24kgs to lose. However I would shed far more in the short months that followed. Interesting to know the Surgeon's I've dealt with in Thailand are nothing short of legendary, not only do they perform surgery multiple times a day, they also work in the public hospital system much like at home and yet they also take the time to teach there craft in local Bangkok Universities to ensure the medical tourism industry continues far into the future for their country. So understandably they are on the go most of the time..

5 SURGERY

The day had finally arrived, the day my life would be drastically changed forever. To put it mildly I was in turmoil and emotionally in two definitive camps, one beyond excited and the other in full on mourning anticipating the end of my yummy food inspired life. Food that I had grown to overindulge in would now not be able to be consumed. Obviously I had that last cheeky meal, I mean really who wouldn't have. Let's face it we were finally in Thailand, so I just had to have a Pad Thai washed down with hot chips not forgetting that beloved Coca Cola, and for desert a chocolate laden waffle the size of a large dinner plate smothered in tropical fruit.

Looking back I think I was actually quite restrained for my last meal it could have been a whole lot worse, trust me. Two weeks leading up to the operation I'd had medical checks to ensure my mortality wasn't on the cards. As the sleeving process is slightly different from country to country in Thailand I wasn't required to partake in any form of liquid diet prior to the surgery. Yet if I was back home I would've been examined to see that my liver had shrunk sufficiently enough to operate due to the liquid only directive. However that said they were also very thorough in Thailand, for instance I had a number of x-rays of my chest and two days prior to the operation I had a gastroscopy (camera inserted down my throat) to inspect the condition of my stomach and to identify any abnormalities. They did in fact find that I had some scaring from a previous ulcer and they were immediately concerned. After a fair amount of discussion among the medical team I received some oral treatment and soon enough I was given clearance by the surgeon to proceed. My operation time was confirmed for later that week. The day before surgery I was contacted and admitted early that evening as I had developed reasonably high blood pressure. The medical team felt I needed normalising prior to undergoing the surgery. After some rest and by the next morning it had improved markedly, so I was given a small breakfast of french toast before the nil by mouth rule would apply. To be fair the nerves had really started to kick in by now, so I didn't even feel like eating much at all. Which is quite amusing when I think about it, I'm pretty sure I regretted that decision very early the next day! Surgery day had finally arrived and it was a bit of a blur thank goodness, it went super fast. The nursing staff kept up with monitoring my blood pressure and trying to reassure me that I was going to be just fine, which helped calm me as my mood often has an affect on my blood pressure. They worked hard on keeping me in good spirits. Before I knew it I was hugging and kissing hubby goodbye, he looked pretty worried but was being upbeat and positive for me. But you just know what was racing through his head when you've been together this long. Fear began to set in and try to pretty much overcome me, especially as they wheeled me into the operating theatre. I remember quickly scanning the room to check that it was similar to the theatres I was used to back home. Fortunately it was, as I think I was probably well past the point of no return by now. The nurses started feverishly hooking me up to all sorts of complex machines with a vast number of tubes. Out of nowhere I felt this strong flood of emotions and started to quietly sob. I think I was coming to realise the enormity of what I'd signed up for, and reality was firmly setting in gripping me. Basically I was freaking out. Guilt hit me too, why had I let myself get so out of control? Why couldn't I just be like all the skinny girls out there and not be so unhealthy and obese. I was so disappointed in myself for having to take this drastic action for all these years of inaction. In a nutshell I was sad that I couldn't beat the food addiction, for whatever reason it hid behind me never letting me win. Emotional damage, comforting food from my Gran whatever excuse I had this just needed to be surgically changed. Out of nowhere two beautiful Thai theatre nurses were above me wiping away my tears and stroking my hair. And one of them bless her, bent down and gently kissed my foreign forehead with a loving smile! That was my last memory of the day, my next memory was waking up in the ward. It was finally over my stomach was now the size of a child's and there was no turning back, not ever! Hubby told me prior to being wheeled in that rather than sit around in the hospital ward obsessing about my fate, he would head off to the mall to check out the electronics goods. Something I definitely didn't need to be there for, later he told me this story. He headed down and walked to the BTS train station. Where he met a French backpacker who kindly helped him board the correct train towards Siam Central. He shopped for a few hours and headed outside to catch the train back which by now was chaos, rush hour had descended on Bangkok and the crowds that spilled out onto the streets were substantial. To make matters worse the heavens had opened and released what appeared like the Niagara Falls upon Siam. He stopped to video it and I can say it was like nothing we'd ever seen before. He was cutting it fine to meet me on the other side and freshly out of surgery. He went to the ticket office and bought a train ticket and after much searching for the right train and platform boarded the wrong train, which headed him further away from me. After a couple of un-recognisable stops he bailed. Now he was really lost and by this stage totally soaked. When weather like this appears in Bangkok the fare charging scooters all take cover, leaving just the cabbies with twice the patronage. The lines were endless. Thinking quickly he started to proposition the scooter drivers who had no clue where he wanted to go and kept pointing towards the sky. Persistence paid off and he managed to negotiate a somewhat expensive wet ride with no raincoat back to the hotel where he could refresh and reattempt the taxi to the hospital. Time was slipping away but thankfully he made up some of the lost time weaving through grid locked traffic similar to swimming through a waterfall with large metal objects coming for you.... Needless to say he did make it back to me before I arrived back to the recovery ward.

6 POST

As I came to I remember looking around with just my eyes as it felt like my head was glued fast to the pillow, heavier than a lump of rock. I reached down and placed my hands gently on the bandages enclosing my stomach, well there it was the proof that I was officially sleeved. I sighed and relaxed for a moment. Now I'm not the best on anesthesia so it felt pretty rough those first few days, all I remember from the surgery is my handsome surgeon (not hubby handsome) telling me that I could not vomit after surgery as that would risk tearing the stitches open. That picture in my head definitely scared me more than I can describe. The reason related back to a surgery a year prior when I had an operation to remove my Gallbladder and then a second operation soon after to scrape my inflamed sinus's. Both times when I came to I spent the next few hours vomiting uncontrollably from the anesthesia. Due to the barrage of questions pre op my surgeon and anesthetist were pretty well aware of my propensity to throw up after surgery and obviously gave me some sort of anti-nausea drugs, because for once I didn't feel nauseated at all, just majorly groggy and really tired. Hubby appeared above me smiling down and asking me if I needed anything, I smiled back but couldn't muster a reply as I had an overpowering urge to fall sleep, and then like the proverbial "one, two, three sleep" of a hypnotist I was out like a light and sleep I did. The next time I opened my eyes I was much more lucid, I noticed that I was hooked up to an intravenous drip to maintain my fluids and to fill me with antibiotics. They had also inserted a catheter prior to surgery for obvious reasons. My surgeon encouraged me to get up and start moving as soon as I could gather the strength. "The sooner the better," he proclaimed in order to speed up the recovery process and to help with the gas pains that sometimes follow stomach surgery. Interestingly when operating on the stomach they fill your abdomen with a gas so they can safely navigate around, it assists the surgeon when removing the majority of your stomach in pieces. I decided to heed his advice and make an attempt to at least sit up and maybe dangle my legs over the bed for starters. So with the help of the nurses I did just that, oh my goodness did my stomach feel sore, it was pretty much the same pain I had felt with the gallbladder removal. It was painful yet horribly awkward to use my stomach muscles, so I used my arms instead to take up the weight and this somewhat comfortably allowed me to move with the least amount of pressure or pain on the abdominal area. Boom, I was upright dangling my feet off the bed and at that very moment I felt the catheter. Joy, what a horrible sensation that is, it's truly the weirdest feeling known, but I do appreciate that there was no other way, except that is for perhaps "Depends adult diapers". I was unable to get myself down onto a toilet seat at this stage so the catheter was a necessity worth enduring, well for now anyway. The nurse did say if I could walk around the ward and practice using my arms more to take the pressure from my stomach, my catheter could be removed, so right there was massive motivation to move forward. My first walk or should I say stand was weird, I was permanently hunched over like I'd dropped a coin on the ground and was bent over looking for it. basically a hunchback. Trying to buffer the pain I took a couple of steps around my recovery room and felt I should sit back down immediately. At this point you face a quandary, your compelled to sit down as you're exhausted but you know you are going to endure pain as you attempt to get back into the bed. So I found myself deliberating over which pain would be the least hurtful, more often than not just standing for a while trying to plan my next painful move. To begin with I felt brave and wanted to exceed the surgeons recovery expectations. I decided to venture out of my room leaning on my IV trolley for support, I headed for the hallway which was a convenient loop past all my new fellow struggling sleever friends and then past the nurses station back into my room. It's a funny sight indeed to see patients shuffling along the ward like emperor penguins around and around, then stopping for a breather and to engage in a quick catch up with fellow patients. Much is discussed in these quick exchanges searching for progress and tips. Mostly we were confirming how we were all feeling. There was some valuable advice being imparted from sleevers that were a couple of days ahead, it was in these catch ups that you realised its not always going to be this way and eventually you would end up looking forward to breaking out of your room to shuffle through the ward amongst the battlers. Some would tell you how they had tried and failed to fool the doctors fudging their water intake, while others where top achievers breezing through and adapting nicely. Even the rebellious who thought they knew better were eventually caught up with if they cut corners. At some point you realised that the professionals told you things for one reason. It was best for you and because it works. Failure to take in water didn't hit the first day or even the second but by the third you would be in dire straights. I spent a fair amount of time sleeping, typically the pain stayed about the same each day, and by day three I could eventually straighten my back up. Now I could impart my knowledge on the newbies! By this stage the nurses and the surgeon were getting a little annoyed with me for not achieving my strictly measured water intake, and in turn I was annoyed right back at them. How can they judge me having not walked this path I thought and really they had no clue, well that was what I was telling myself anyway. There were two water intake road blocks for me. The first was that you literally could only sip water in tiny wee amounts and the second was that before this operation I absolutely loathed water. I really don't know how I survived for 49 years without it but I just did, I could literally go for weeks without drinking any water so this was almost akin to mission impossible for me. Obviously the surgeon knew what he was talking about and could sense my resistance, so we struck a deal. I could flavour the water and they would take out the IV and closely monitor my water intake. He warned me that he would know pretty much straight away if I wasn't meeting the water intake requirement. He said he would have no hesitation in hooking me up to the drip again should I not comply and would effectively keep me incarcerated for a lot longer than the prescribed amount of recovery time. So we agreed and it was gratefully removed. I was free to push myself along independently and sipped away constantly. I can tell you also that knowing my meals were coming three times a day helped me to cope, because the stop drinking rule that applies to meals thirty mins prior to eating was certainly some welcomed relief to this girl that just doesn't do water. My one saving grace was that I had found from talking with the other patients that the addition of sugar free protein drops into my bottle turned the bland water into something I could actually consume, which proves once more how important it is to collaborate with your gastric sleeve peers. What do you know it actually worked for me, another Hallelujah moment. With my water issue somewhat under control, my stomach was adapting quite nicely and by now included soft foods which I detail in the next chapter. My external incisions were also healing quite nicely and after the five days I was given the green light to leave the hospital and head back to the hotel to recover. This was exciting news for me but also a mixed bag of emotions, some of empowerment others about letting go of the close medical attention. I could not wait to shop for my own food though, good food that is. I'm pretty confident that they make hospital food taste pretty bad for one reason, its so you leave. The surgeon cleared me to step it up and now introduce pretty much normal foods into diet, like grilled meats and vegetables. He warned me to stay away from any form of bread at this time because the stomach takes longer to adjust to certain carbohydrates. Luckily for me we were in Bangkok so there were many food establishments grilling chicken skewers and selling delicious steamed vegetables. To put the food portion size into context at this early stage, I could have in one sitting a small bite of a chicken skewer, and half a small broccoli floret (not a head) and that was it I was done, full as a dam about to burst its banks. Wow unbelievable, I don't think hubby could quite believe it either, before seeing it with his very own eyes he thought they just pretended they had operated on people and took the cash. But here it was the undeniable proof. It dawned on him that I was now definitely one cheap date.

7 NEW REGIME

As I mentioned earlier my surgeon had explained in detail that I could regain my weight if I was not diligently following the new eating guidelines. He cautioned that I would have approximately one year to adjust, which he likened fondly to the "honeymoon period." Obviously this honeymoon did not include the better aspects like champagne and romance. He was enlightening me to the fact that there was no possible way I would physically be able to eat very much at all for the first year at least. So in his eyes this was like a gift, now I would be armed with a decent amount of time to change, and reprioritise my vast collection of unhealthy eating habits. He has performed a lot of surgery's and monitored post op many thousands of patients. It's all he does no cosmetics, no skin removal just sleeves. His experience makes him pretty knowledgeable when it comes to both eating with a newly sleeved stomach and then maintaining it into the future. As a consequence you may find his advice somewhat different to the advice of others, especially if you compared notes from that of a typical western medical patient. Undertaking a little of your own research about gastric sleeve surgery will produce a pre and post op diet process more than likely set out as follows: Pre op will consist of 3-4 weeks fasting and dieting with only meal replacement shakes and salads etc. to decrease the liver size. Post op has 4 main stages: Stage 1: Clear fluids in the first 2 weeks including water, herbal tea, clear broth and sugar free apple juice, you can then introduce skimmed milk, smooth clear soups and meal replacement drinks. Stage 2: Pureed foods weeks 3 to 4 once you can tolerate liquids, start on pureed foods, liquidised meat, fish stew, eggs and thick creamy soups. You must include in your meals 60 - 80 grams of protein a day. Stage 3: Soft foods from week 5 -6 you can start adding soft foods including minced meats, fish, cottage cheese, cooked veggies etc again you must consume at least 60 - 80 grams of protein a day and drink 1.5 to 2 litres of water per day. Stage 4 : Normal but reduced diet weeks 6 - 8 From my experience and speaking with other patients they say that after six weeks resuming a normal solid food diet is totally achievable. Your new sleeve will by then allow you to eat almost any type or texture of food. That said Surgeon's commonly advise you to avoid foods high in fat or sugar such as biscuits, chips, ice cream, sweets, white bread, rice, fibrous vegetables and chewy meats. You are instructed to consume at least 60 - 80 grams of protein in a given day and drink approximately1.5 to 2 litres of water per day. I can't stress enough to you how important water is as I developed a hernia from blocking up and becoming constipated. My body tried to adjust to a whole new way of processing small amounts without the enormous fat intake it was used to, there's more on this subject later in the book. My surgeon had carefully reiterated what he expected from me after the surgery. It went something like this: Firstly we would be on a diet of clear broth a day out of surgery and that we should learn to sip water constantly throughout the day. This would help to keep us hydrated and assist in having our drips removed. The water and food also assists us in jump starting our stomach whilst we would go through the intensive healing process. We were discouraged from using a straw to drink through as there was the possibility you would create excessive gas in the stomach and in addition we could take in more liquid than our stomach could accept at that point. So straws were definitely out. By day three or four depending on how we were coping, we were served a soft omelet and broth which we ate for the duration of our stay in the hospital. He instructed us to slowly introduce real foods straight back into our lives by day five post op. We were repeatedly instructed to chew, chew, chew our food at least 40 times before finally swallowing it. Of course this was problematic for most of us as we realised that we had been a little too hasty when inhaling our meals in our pre sleeve era. The chew chew chew theory was probably the hardest of all the bad habits to get under control. At least for me anyway. I would picture the stitches in my stomach opening up and eventually I would adapt to the repetition helping it to stick with me. This is not similar to the west I hear you say, but on closer observation there is a similarity, chewing forty times a mouthful soon turns your food into something that resembles machine processed food. This produces a second benefit, it teaches the undisciplined eater like me to slow it down from day one and turns food into a digestible easier to process slurry full of absorbable nutrients. I told you this guy was brilliant. Drinking and then eating in the same sitting was also a definitive no, it became pretty clear that it was either one or other. There had to be a period of at least half an hour between liquids and solid meals. So thinking ahead and planning out the day became an effective way to survive. We too were instructed to consume at least 60 - 80 grams of protein a day like our normal western counterparts. The protein portion was to be consumed first off the plate, before anything else as this would give us the feeling of fullness a lot quicker. Interestingly related to the protein and due to the upheaval your body endures many woman lose large handfuls of their hair in the months following surgery, so fearing hair loss this protein first method made a lot of sense to me. We were not to overeat at all. We also needed to stop eating before we even started to feel full, now this rule was tough at first as I didn't really even feel hunger pangs at all. This rule went hand in hand with chew, chew, chew because if you obeyed this rule and chewed, you were forced to slow down enough to actually hear your stomach telling you that you've had quite enough. Failure to hear your stomach resulted in sharp pains and nausea. Too much sharp pain and I got to thinking I would stretch what was left of my stomach. So I learned to stop. In those early stages my mind was still thinking a bit too much like old large portion me. I mistakenly thought I could prepare and get through about the same size meals as I had prior to the surgery, which by the way was now a physical impossibility and most of it would go into the garbage. Another fun side effect is that your body finds a way to signal you that you're full. I along with a lot of other sleevers developed what you might call a tick, not the insect type, more the repeated reaction resulting from eating too much type. So every time I started feeling near full and this happens to this very day nearly two years on, I quietly let out a burp, at this point I should put down the utensils and stop eating. If I choose to ignore this first sign my nose then starts to drip like I've got a cold, and if I really turn it up and rebel completely against the signs I start sneezing uncontrollably! I mean what the hell is that, every single time like clock-work I have a built in signal. Trust me if I overeat this absolutely happens to me, mind blown! The surgeon also didn't want us to get our protein requirements through any form of protein shake, He felt they were more likely than not to contain other unwanted things like sweeteners which would reduce your early progress. He instead wanted us eating high protein rich naturally found foods that would help us obtain the daily recommended intake. Like fresh cut meats and leafy green vegetables. As he put it "We get better nutrients this way" and it was a more realistic method to retrain our eating habits. He explained that failure comes easier if we rely on something like shakes three times a day, as we would need to reintroduce real food at some point in the future without having learnt the best method of adopting good food choices. He thought that we were not designed to live on this type of processed sustenance anyway. Another piece of great advice was that if we were going to cook ourselves a meal we should if possible buy the best cut available, like Wagyu eye fillet, as it normally melts in your mouth, its easier to break down and the quantity would be in a word, miniscule. He also said something to me that just stuck, he said "You have so few bites of food available now that you should make them the best you possibly can, go for taste every time not quantity and don't ever waste a bite eating rubbish as you wont have room for something tasty." This little comment helped me so much psychologically, I mean lets face it I'd gotten here from piling it in, now it was about taste, and this my friends made my transitional journey down the scales much much easier and actually more enjoyable. It really resonated with me and to this day I still try not to waste precious small bites with empty calories and tasteless foods. I guess he did retrain me after all! Wow, what a legend. Walking got easier and easier around the hotel, there was by now a large steadfast group of sleevers who would walk together and catch up on the issues we faced. We encouraged each other on the small wins, like one of us having a catheter removed on day two post op. Although we had all endured the same operation by the same surgeon our healing and coping mechanisms were vastly different. I truly believe you can't compare this journey with anyone else's, we are all uniquely different. So its great to talk to others but don't get me wrong you can do your mind a lot of damage if you start comparing your weight loss progress, reflux and what your stomach can and cannot handle to the person down the hall. So here we were hubby and I back at our hotel to recuperate for a couple of weeks before heading to our new home in Queensland Australia. There was a seven eleven right next to the hotel so we ventured there to see what I could stock up on as I didn't have the energy to venture too far in the searing heat of the tropics at this point. I bought low fat no sugar yoghurt and edam cheese for my lunches. Breakfast was complementary as part of the hotel package so there was the usual big buffet which was always popular. Picture this though, a long line of newly sleeved patients at the egg station ordering their one egg in the normal variety of ways, scrambled, omelet with cheese, or eggs over easy. It was a good start for us to help get our protein intake up for the day and everyone was rather excited about it for the first three days or so, after that everyone got utterly sick of them. So you could work out pretty quickly who were the sleevers and how far they'd come by scanning the restaurant at breakfast. They would be the ones taking ridiculously small bites and looked to be in obvious pain. It was not physical pain that was registering on their faces it was the realisation that they couldn't eat anywhere near what they were used to anymore. It was in some ways quite amusing but also sad as we were all mourning in our own quiet way. What have we done became the most common thought amongst us, especially in those first few weeks post op. It's a lot to comprehend one day you are eating whatever you want receiving your euphoric fix for the day, and now here you are barely able to eat a quarter of your one egg omelet. There was undoubtedly a fair amount of wastage as the sleevers slowly adjusted. Dinner was pretty much the same every night in Bangkok, charcoaled chicken skewers. They were tasty, high in protein and convenient. The surgeons words kept ringing in my head, eat protein and don't waste your bites, so I didn't and felt better for it. Hubby thought we should do some touristy things to get to know the place which I happily agreed to. So on day two from being discharged from the hospital I decided it would be a great idea to go to a Thai cooking class in the early afternoon followed by a show in the evening. My sister had visited Thailand a couple of times and highly recommended a cooking class. So I know what you're thinking - its probably not the best time to do this but we didn't think we would ever be back, so it was now or never. Although I kept pushing my cooked meals onto my husband because I couldn't make a dent in the five courses I can say it was the best day we had in Bangkok. Jay the chef at Silom cooking school was unbelievably knowledgeable, uber talented and really funny. We cooked up a storm and Peter our tour guide picked us up from the cooking class to go and enjoy the must see show Siam Niramet which was outstanding. Peter was one of the nicest people we had the good fortune to meet in Thailand he always made our outings meaningful with his immense knowledge of everything Thai. After the show he transported us back to the hotel and on the way he played James Blunt's "You're Beautiful" which became carpool karaoke learning and singing the words in Thai, to this day every time we hear this song hubby and I will attempt to sing it in Thai, it warms our heart. The hotel staff were excellent, in particular we have fond memories of a lovely Thai man named

Jit he treated us with such kindness and everyday would help us get around safely, taking a genuine interest in our wellbeing whilst we stayed at the hotel. Deep down you knew that they struggled through life like a lot of us at times, but their situation seemed a lot harder to pull out of. Regardless of their situation whatever they faced outside of the hotel it never showed. They would do anything to make your time in Thailand more memorable. It truly was a sad day for us leaving Bangkok, besides the fact that I had undergone this life changing surgery, it was the lovely people we left behind that made it tough to leave. Two years on and we booked in again this time for skin removal surgery and believe it or not Jit remembered us like an old friend! We packed our things and off we headed to our next adventure.

8 COPING

Over the preceding months the weight truly melted away much like the preverbal iceberg floating in the Caribbean. The pace was astounding and within a very short time I looked like a new person, I really didn't feel like a new person or much different at all for that matter, I just looked a whole lot thinner externally and it was now registering in the mirror. Years of hiding behind things and feeling ashamed of who I'd become would be difficult to change psychologically, long into the future. My clothing choices always for some reason were two sizes too big, and as the excess skin started to appear I went from covering fat to covering excess wrinkles. So I had old me thinking in a new me body. Hubby was excited for me even venturing out to buy me some new clothes on my way down the scales. Which soon proved he had taken his shot a little bit early as they ended up fitting for a couple of weeks before being unwearable. We settled into our new life in the Gold Coast it was similar in a lot of ways to home. We rented a two bedroom apartment, while we searched for something decent to buy. Hubby landed a job and was gone most days so I spent a good chunk of my time trying to come to grips with the size of these unusually tiny meals and how to make them as tasty as possible. I weighed in at home once a week, losing just under two kilo's each time measured. I began to notice that I was getting into the groove of adjusting to the minuscule portions and soon realised that for the first time in a long time I had this weight thing pretty much under control. It appeared with a sleeve to be a lot easier than anything I had attempted in the diet scene ever before. It made perfect sense now that restricting the size of my meals to extra small, drinking water and removing the hunger pangs would leave no option but send my addiction packing. I knew deep down this sort of progress would not have been possible with out the sleeve. I had hit just on 90kg by the time I left Thailand which amounted to about 10kg in a little over two weeks. I left Thailand and settled into the more familiar food choices of home pretty effortlessly and my diet at that stage consisted of for breakfast, a half a scrambled egg with grated cheese and chopped chive sprinkles with a tablespoon of taste free protein powder for good measure. For lunch I normally cooked a small chicken thigh with some more protein powder sprinkled over the top, and at this point would only be able to consume about 20grams before I would let out a burp which rendered me full. I would then put the left over chicken aside for dinner with cooked or raw vegetables. In between meals I would have a teaspoon of Greek yogurt and sip on high protein milk shakes to try and reach the recommended daily protein intake. As you can imagine the weight had no chance hanging on with such a reduction in portion. Before I knew it I was at 85kg and now just four weeks out of surgery. My clothing started to look ridiculous and I became awestruck at just how fast the process to lose weight had become. You may wonder about my desire for food, let me tell you that it was gone, however those habits formed over 48 years to graze regularly all day still existed. Some strange urge in me expected the fridge to be opened regularly, the preparation to be done and to have food in front of me at all times, whether this was simply the fear of missing out or perhaps some other reason it was tough adjusting. My eyes had not registered to my stomach limits or needs and my mind was not aligned with either. I started shopping for new clothes but not too many as I knew they too would be soon rendered surplus. As I reached 83kg I remember feeling I could step it up a bit. At this moment I crossed the line from weight reduction for healthiness into becoming scales obsessed. Something switched in me and now I wanted to lose more, so I searched for an App to see if it could help me start to count what little calories I consumed. "My Fitness Pal" was to become my second best or worst tool in weight loss depending on how you looked at it. The first being of course my sleeve. I'd agreed on the advice of my Doctor to settle on 800Kj per day to bring me down to the desired weight. I was now able to stay on track measuring the energy going in and weighing everything I ate. Rating packets became my new existence. As an aside I'd been encouraged to do this a long time ago by the more healthier people around me, but this time I took to it without the condescending feelings of a bygone era like a duck to water. I would record all manner of data including my fat burn through daily exercise like doing the house work and long walks on the beach. I clocked up on average 10,000 steps a day and refused to go to bed without achieving my walking goal. Now that I was fully in the swing of it I dipped below the 80's to 79kg's and was thinking I should probably slow down a little, but I hadn't seen this size for a very long time or been here since my early teens. It felt unbelievable, something that I had long ago accepted as just not possible. As I crept towards the 70kg's I kept on with diligently entering my calories and exercise burn into the phone app. The danger with this method is that you can feel better about life if you beat the target so coming in under 800Kj felt great, that's when things start getting wobbly soon turns to less is more and in this case more weight loss. By week twelve I breezed on past the 70kg's, not a problem. Still consuming the same heavily filled protein diet, occasionally heading out for dinner at the local surf club. I would order a large steak and when it arrived I ate about two mouthfuls, wrapped it up and placed it quietly into my handbag for later. I would consume the same piece of steak over the next two days making beef sandwiches and cheesy wraps for both lunch and dinner, so I managed to get up to six meals out of it, which is just nuts. I reached the 60kgs mark by week twenty four and to be fair I looked pretty gaunt, almost sickly thin. Excess skin had begun to show up on my thighs, bottom, arms and stomach, which really bothered me. I finally hit the high fifties and plateaued. Wow I thought is this what it felt like for my skinny friends, I was super excited to wake up and get dressed each day into something that didn't resemble a yurt. By this stage I had obviously changed my thinking towards the outside because now I wanted to be out and about in the sunshine instead of in the confines of home watching all those sad sack talk shows. I feel that my hubby if asked would've said I had pushed a bit too far and had now crossed the line, into becoming disturbingly obsessed with my new weight. Now more than ever before in my life I wanted to keep on losing. Madness. I knew I looked unsightly but I really needed to prove to myself just how far I could go having these tools. My thinking again wasn't exactly right, only this time at the other end of the scales from XXL with all its personal toll to XXS and all its obsession. Fortunately for me though my body just would not lose another pound so I sat bony as a school kid at 57 kgs and from then on I have never ever managed to increase my weight, I have simply maintained this weight. Family members worried I had got terminally sick, and hubby was really anxious as he'd never seen me at this size, ever. Even all those years ago when we were teenagers dating. This was a massive deal for me but I didn't comprehend how it would affect him either. He had now done a 360 and rather than sell me on eating well he pleaded me to stop tracking my calories on the phone App. I agreed in principle but just couldn't bring myself to switch the darn thing off, I was hooked and basically fibbed to him saying I no longer used it. Not my proudest but that's obsession I guess. Looking back I was at that time bordering on sliding off the cliff and into a full on eating disorder. The calorie intake goal was now achievable for the first time in my life so on I went trying to beat the app inputs, more steps less intake. This could've ended badly I and everyone around me just knew it. About the fourth month out my Mum and Dad came over to visit us. One of the days I confided in Mum about how hubby was feeling about the darn App and how I couldn't actually switch it off. She just looked at me with that worried look in her eyes and said "You are too skinny," she followed it up with "look you have done amazingly, but that's enough now." I knew that look from my mother, so

I had to get a grip on it rather than it on me. Lets face it I had just battled the morbidly obese demon and won with the help of my new sleeve. I did not ever imagine or want to be at the other end of the spectrum fighting a different demon. So I resolved to stop and that's what I did. Over the next couple of days I closed the App. My disorder also presented other issues because by now I had found a large lump just above my pelvis bone. Naturally all sorts of things rush through your mind, the worst being cancer. So hubby put me on a plane pretty much the same day to get an appointment with my doctor and to visit our son whom I was missing terribly. I managed to see my Doctor the very next day and on viewing the protrusion he suspected it was an inguinal hernia, but waisted no time checking to see that it wasn't something else like a form of benign tumour. The normal barrage of tests were carried out, MRI's, CT scans, bloodwork and the likes, as usual he was very thorough. A few days later and as he suspected it was thankfully a hernia that needed to be attended to by another surgeon. I had lost a staggering amount of weight, approximately 40 kg's of fat. So understandably I was extremely boney. Meaning the thick layer of cushioning fat all over my body was now gone. I felt the cold, the bed everything was more present without my old protective layer of fat to absorb the knocks. As a result it soon had revealed my collar bones, rib cage, hip bones and even my knobby knees. My breasts had shrunk away to tiny little B cups. As I waited for my surgery which was scheduled for about six weeks time I stayed with my son for a good chunk of it. Once the operation was competed I headed back to Queensland to resume our now normal empty nesters lifestyle. One morning a few months later while taking a shower I felt another lump this time it was sticking out the side of my left breast, good grief I thought not something else. The fact that I was bordering gaunt had revealed a lump that would possibly have been hidden for quite some time under a few layers. Now it was out it scared both hubby and I terribly. Once again I was back onboard a plane as quick as possible and off to see the doctor. More tests and biopsy's revealed that this time around in fact it was benign. I remember the day vividly and was pretty thankful and relieved that's for sure. While I was there my Doctor had requested a retest and review of my bloodwork along with my levels. He informed me that I was in really good shape (other than the lump) which was a welcome relief. To be on the safe side l was scheduled in for more surgery to remove the lump just in case it decided to change its status from benign to malignant at some point in the future. After surgery and recovery I once again left for Queensland, this time it was for good. I was now fully into the maintenance phase of my sleeve so by this stage the Doctor had advised me to increase my calories to 1200Kj per day. Helping me enjoy a longer healthy lifestyle without further reducing my size. He also requested that I add more vegetables and fruit into my diet, something I had generally ignored and always struggled with pre sleeve. Apart from my new Kj target my doctor also refused to agree with any kind of Ketosis (low carb) diet and felt that losing the weight was not going to be one of my problems in the future. He couldn't understand why I'd even entertain such an unhealthy diet choice which comes from discussions in a large part of the sleever community. Many insist we follow the various Keto type diets, some even get a bit nasty and troll Facebooker's defending their one sided advice. This however was his advice for me. (understandably you may have quite different guidance from your own doctor) That said though this is my personal journey offered to you as a biography, not that rigid just an example on how I got through along with all the choices and advice that I took. For me even from the beginning it worked great. Totally void of the regimented ketosis method. It was difficult for me to even get close to the 1200Kj a day, so most of the time I would land short at about 1000Kj. Strangely like my old dress size that now looked like an enormous amount of food to me. Here is how a typical day looked like now: One scrambled or poached egg, a tablespoon of baked beans or spaghetti and half a piece of toast with butter and a small piccolo coffee with full cream milk. A snack would be a ham slice rolled up with cheese, cucumber, tomato and a wheat cracker. For lunch I would cook up a small chicken thigh, around 50 grams and have this with a small salad. I would finish off eating a piece of fruit of either one slice of watermelon, a handful of blueberries or a quarter of a cup of mango these seemed to be my favorites. Dinner would normally be much the same as lunch with some sort of cooked meat or poultry along with a salad or vegetables. Sometimes depending on the time of the month a small potato was added in. At this time it was still the same for me as it was before the sleeve surgery, I was ravenous all day for about 2-3 days and craved anything sweet like chocolate. So of course I would indulge a little as my sleeve could only tolerate a small bite. Obviously this was quite a step down in quantity from before the sleeve, as I could devour a large king size block in about two sittings at this time of the month! As time zoomed on past from my original sleeve surgery I became plagued with constipation, which from all accounts seems to be a common factor amongst the sleever community. To be blatantly honest I was clearly not consuming enough water and in addition to the lack of water I was eating too much protein first in my meals. This would in turn fill me up and not leave any wiggle room for vegetables, fruit, fibre or good oils that could assist me in passing the waste. So eventually my stomach ground to a complete halt and the solids backed up. With all the increased pressure now being applied to force a bowel movement and in order to pass the somewhat rock hard waste there was an unfortunate side effect. As mentioned above the weakened area in my abdominal wall opened on up and the inguinal hernia popped on out. So it's important for anyone thinking of undertaking this journey to know how to keep movements actually moving. I would fully recommend that you discover the best foods that keep you on the run as it were, you will be far more at ease in the long term. For me I have introduced in somewhat small amounts: Prune juice, bran, chilli, pear and more water. By month six my hair had started to really thin out and then even fall out. This was rough as I'd always had very fine hair and managed to block most drains with just how much it shed. It always replenished fine enough back then and was long and beautifully healthy. Not post sleeve though, now it was devastatingly light and thin. I would best describe it as "see through hair" When I looked in the mirror I could see through it to the back. So I had to accept the change and have it restyled short. My hair prior to cutting was about half way down my back and after they had layered it into a bob just above my shoulders. Hair was a great way for me to hide my overly rounded face, so I'd leave my hair down to cover it, but now that it was cut short I couldn't hide a thing. From my research and talking to my Doctor hair loss can be attributed to a lack of protein and nutrients being absorbed. Another big contributor thought to be attributed to hair loss is the anesthetic process from all the surgery's. I have read countless articles on this subject along with their recommendations including having biotin. All I can say is make sure your protein intake is high along with your fibre, vitamins and minerals. That said I personally think sleeve surgery affects us all differently. As I've read the testimonies of many others doing all the above and more yet still their hair loss is uncontrollable and then others who don't lose their hair at all....

9 NEW LIFE

As I'm now finally where I longed to be for so much of my adult life, I thought it necessary to put into descriptive words my thoughts and feelings having completed the surgery and living a somewhat now healthier existence. One of my reasons for going through with the surgery was to feel better about who I am, I can tell you that its pretty surreal, adapting to the new me is the bit that takes time especially after so many years of food abuse hiding behind clothing tents and full bodied hair. It can also be a bit like finally reaching a personal goal with some much needed external assistance and then thinking what's next to tackle. Yes I have changed externally and definitely can say I get a lot of nice complements on how good I look. Would I do this all over again knowing what I know now, the short answer is "Hell yes!" Would I have changed anything that would've made my journey easier, perhaps avoiding the causes of my hernia for one. I'm still confident that anyone going to go ahead with this type of surgery will find they will reach their pinnacle regardless of the methods used. Inevitably you will be made to take on some form of instruction to get through, keeping in the back of your mind some of the challenges I faced will hold you in good stead. The size of the stomach is the key here, it's drastically reduced so really it comes down to adopting those methods that get you through easier and marching onwards to a better healthier more vibrant you. I have reached the conclusion that I should've had this surgery undertaken twenty years earlier saving myself an enormous amount of wasted time and cash not just for the added need for skin removal surgery which I elected for some fourteen months later, but all those years of diet anxiety, extreme food bills and stupid fast food addictions. My 30 year old self would've appreciated the surgery for good reason a lot sooner and that's for certain. To be blunt there was no real way for me to have ever beaten my addictions or eating disorders or whatever label I gave it, other than through receiving the sleeve surgery. I believe that people are all very different some have no trouble keeping weight at bay, others have no trouble carrying a lot of excess. I'm not either of these things as I care a little too much about what others think of me. Hubby says that he didn't care either way I was and that "I shouldn't give a shite" about what others think anyhow. He thinks I should just be content with who I am. So in reality because I couldn't manage weight contentment as he puts it, the sleeve became the best and probably the only realistic option for me. You and others around you are probably quite different to me in regards to your thoughts on weight and how others see you. And if you truly have an ounce of self-control, can enjoy exercise then a healthy lifestyle without a sleeve is still the best option hands down. But for those of us that aren't able to deal with the addiction all I can say is thank God for the surgeons throughout the earth that can now sleeve us. It gives us a shot of what normal is like. I want to say a big Thank You to my doctor and my surgeon and all the wonderful nurses because now I've finally been healed. I hope I've answered some of your more pressing questions about what sleeving actually feels like from the pain to the coping with a reduced stomach and eventually onto the healthy lifestyle that is waiting for you to arrive. If you would like to ask anything about my journey you can contact me on my twitter handle @Sleeverdiva

10 DOMINO

When the body changes from a sleeve and rest assured it does perhaps not as dramatically as mine did, your epithelial tissue (skin) can't shrink back or resize like it used to when you were younger. To put in into context you are left with a size 24 skin covering on a size 10 frame. You may be thinking good grief and rightly so, weight gain is one thing to tackle but to have this sort of damage on the other side of it isn't what you're expecting. Was I in for a big shock I really thought I would be resilient enough to dodge this one, but alas here I was looking like a Sharpei puppy. As you can imagine I was up for the challenge and tried in vain to moisturise, exercise and massage my skin back to a previous time in history. A more skin forgiving bounce back time that is. Whatever method I tried it had little to no effect. Eventually one must accept defeat when nothing else is working and begin the process all over again this time in preparation for a surgical skin removal procedure. Research, quotes and consensus would need to be completed. I'm happy to report that I'm sitting here writing this book in Da Nang Vietnam, having left from Thailand three weeks ago and now nicely recovering from my cosmetic skin removal surgery. If you're interested in knowing the complete story of skin surgery, the pain, the results and the things to avoid, My next book "Sleeve outer layer XS TO XL" will document the whole process, pre op appointments, after surgery care, the best way's I found to deal with scaring and once again it captures it all. I will once more go into detail as to what you should expect if you're considering this form of surgery to help you resize your stubborn outer layer. Hope you can join me on a journey amongst the pages, and this time my Mum accompany me to partake in a surgical adventure undergoing skin removal surgery at the very same time! Until then safe travels.

ABOUT THE AUTHOR

I am in my late forty's and married with one fantastic, beautifully compassionate son. I now live a life filled with adventure and can confess that I waisted far too much of it in a weight related struggle. I do things that were not possible before surgery. The old me wasn't ever going to live a fulfilled life so I'm thankful everyday for the surgery that saved me.

Thank you for reading my story and I hope you are inspired to find your happy place!

www.ingramcontent.com/pod-product-compliance
Lightning Source LLC
Chambersburg PA
CBHW020551220526
45463CB00006B/2265